The Mediterranean *Diet cookbook for* Pregnant Women

60+ Delicious and Nutrient-Rich Recipes for a Healthy Pregnancy Journey

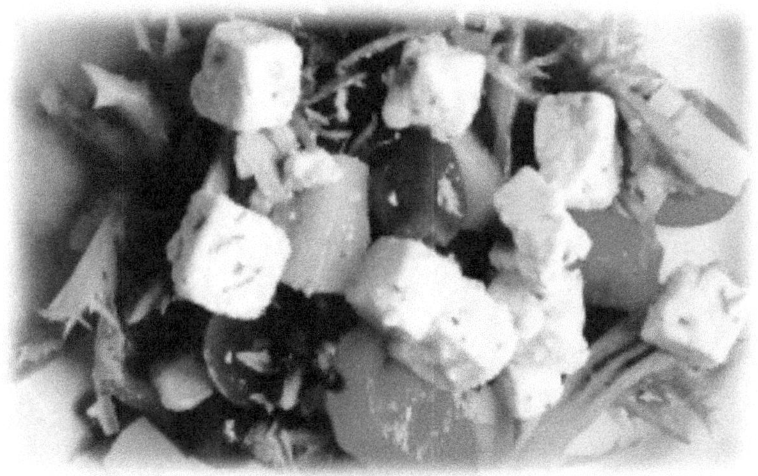

MARRIES-ESTHER LLOYD

Copyright © 2023 by MARRIES-ESTHER LLOYD

Disclaimer: The information provided in this book is intended to be accurate and reliable. However, the author and the publisher cannot be held liable for any errors, omissions, or consequences resulting from using the information in this book.

TABLE OF CONTENT

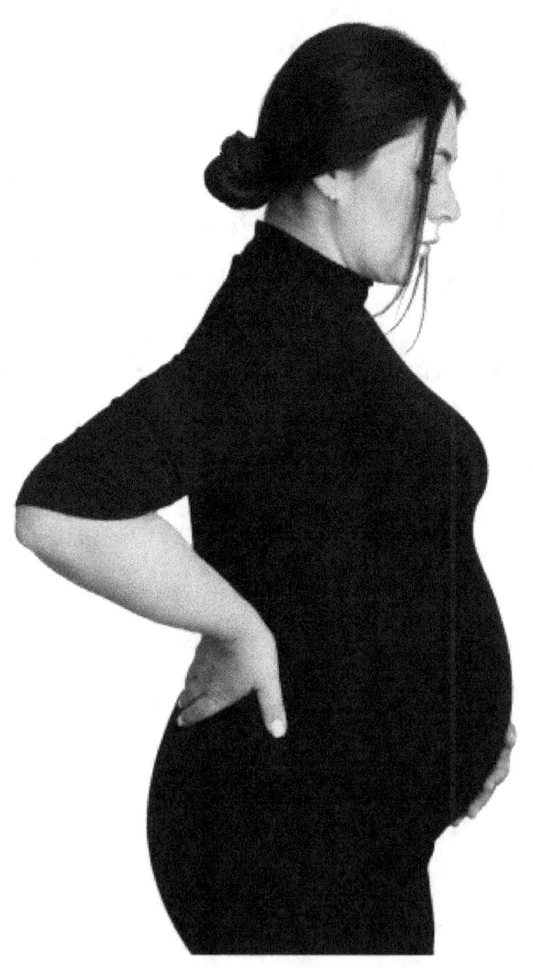

A Mediterranean meal plan for pregnant women is based on the traditional dietary patterns of countries bordering the Mediterranean Sea, such as Greece, Italy, Spain, and southern France.

It emphasizes a wide variety of nutrient-rich foods, which can provide numerous benefits during pregnancy. Here's what you should know about the Mediterranean meal plan for pregnant women and its benefits:

Key Components of a Mediterranean Meal Plan:

1. *Fresh Fruits and Vegetables:* The diet is rich in colorful fruits and vegetables, providing essential vitamins, minerals, and antioxidants for fetal development and maternal health.

2. *Whole Grains:* Whole grains like whole wheat, brown rice, and quinoa offer complex carbohydrates and fiber, promoting steady energy and digestive health.

3. *Lean Proteins:* Lean protein sources like poultry, fish, legumes, and occasional red meat are included, offering essential amino acids for both mother and baby.

4. *Healthy Fats:* Olive oil, nuts, and seeds are staples, providing monounsaturated fats that support heart health and aid in the absorption of fat-soluble vitamins.

5. *Dairy and Dairy Alternatives:* Greek yogurt, cheese, and occasional milk are sources of calcium and probiotics, while lactose-free or plant-based alternatives are suitable for those with lactose intolerance.

6. *Fatty Fish:* The diet encourages the consumption of fatty fish like salmon and sardines, which provide omega-3 fatty acids important for the development of the baby's brain and nervous system.

7. *Legumes:* Beans, lentils, and chickpeas are a good source of protein, fiber, and folate, an essential nutrient during pregnancy.

8. *Herbs and Spices:* Mediterranean herbs and spices, such as oregano, thyme, and garlic, add flavor without the need for excess salt.

Benefits of Following a Mediterranean Meal Plan during Pregnancy:

1. *Nutrient-Rich:* The Mediterranean diet is rich in vitamins, minerals, and antioxidants, providing a well-rounded array of nutrients essential for a healthy pregnancy.

2. *Heart Health:* The inclusion of monounsaturated fats from olive oil, nuts, and seeds supports cardiovascular health, which is important during pregnancy.

3. *Fiber:* High-fiber foods like fruits, vegetables, and whole grains help alleviate constipation and promote regular digestion.

4. *Omega-3 Fatty Acids:* Fatty fish in the diet supplies essential omega-3 fatty acids that are important for the development of the baby's brain and vision.

5. *Healthy Weight Management:* The diet encourages balanced portions and a variety of nutrient-dense foods, which can help manage weight gain during pregnancy.

6. *Gestational Diabetes Prevention:* The Mediterranean diet's emphasis on whole grains and low-glycemic foods can help reduce the risk of gestational diabetes.

7. *Reduced Risk of Birth Defects:* The Mediterranean diet is naturally high in folate, which is important for preventing neural tube defects.

8. *Lowered Risk of Preterm Birth:* Some studies suggest that a Mediterranean diet might be associated with a lower risk of preterm birth.

9. *Reduction in Inflammation:* The diet's anti-inflammatory components may help reduce the risk of chronic inflammation during pregnancy.

10. *Enjoyable and Sustainable:* The Mediterranean diet is known for its delicious and diverse foods, making it easier for pregnant women to adhere to a healthy eating plan.

It's important to note that while the Mediterranean diet offers many health benefits during pregnancy, individual dietary needs may vary.

It's advisable for pregnant women to consult with a healthcare provider or registered dietitian to ensure that their dietary plan meets their specific nutritional requirements and health conditions.

Additionally, any dietary changes during pregnancy should be discussed with a healthcare professional.

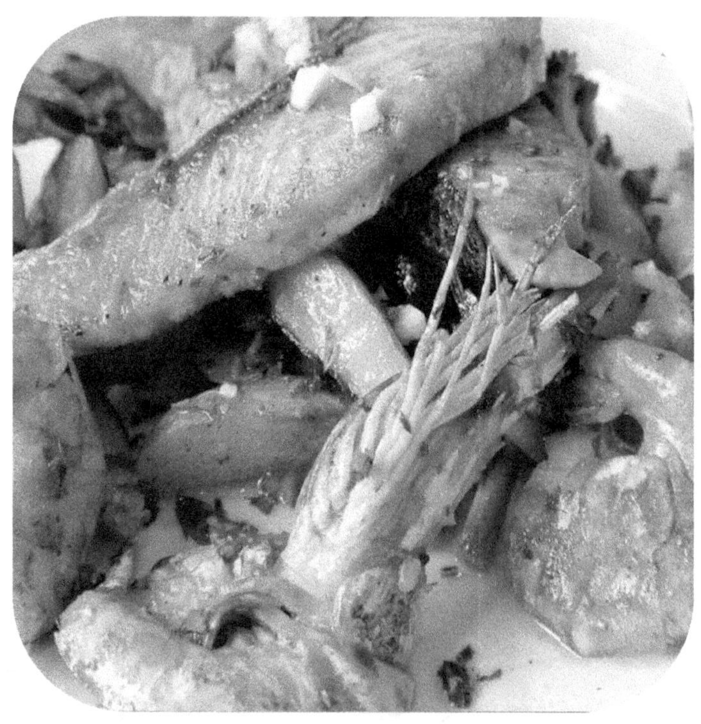

Here's an outline of a Mediterranean Break Fast diet suitable for pregnancy, along with ingredients and instructions:

1. *Mediterranean Greek Yogurt Parfait*

   Ingredients:

   * Greek yogurt (full-fat or low-fat)

   * Fresh berries (blueberries strawberries, or raspberries)

   * Honey

   * Chopped nuts (e.g., walnuts or almonds)

   * Whole-grain granola

   Instructions:

   1. In a bowl or glass, layer Greek yogurt.

   2. Add fresh berries and drizzle honey on top.

   3. Sprinkle with chopped nuts and whole-grain granola.

   4. Enjoy as a nutritious and filling breakfast.

2. *Mediterranean Vegetable Omelette*

   Ingredients:

   * Eggs

* Spinach or kale

* Red bell pepper (diced)

* Onion (diced)

* Feta cheese (crumbled)

* Extra-virgin olive oil

* Herbs (like basil or oregano)

Instructions:

1. Sauté vegetables in olive oil until tender.

2. Beat eggs with herbs and pour over the veggies.

3. Cook until the eggs are set, then sprinkle with feta cheese.

3. *Mediterranean Smoothie Bowl*

* *Ingredients:*

* Greek yogurt

* Mixed berries

* Banana (sliced)

* Honey

* Granola

* Chopped nuts

Instructions:

1. Blend Greek yogurt and mixed berries into a smoothie.

2. Pour into a bowl and top with banana slices, honey, granola, and chopped nuts.

4. *Mediterranean Shakshuka*

Ingredients:

* Eggs

* Tomatoes (diced)

* Bell peppers (diced)

* Onion (chopped)

* Garlic (minced)

* Paprika and cumin (for seasoning)

* Fresh parsley (chopped)

Instructions:

1. Sauté onions, garlic, and bell peppers in olive oil.

2. Add diced tomatoes and spices, then simmer.

3. Crack eggs into the tomato mixture, cover, and cook until the eggs are set.

4. Garnish with fresh parsley before serving.

5. *Mediterranean Avocado Toast*

Ingredients:

* Whole-grain bread

* Ripe avocado

* Tomato slices

* Feta cheese

* Extra-virgin olive oil

* Fresh basil leaves

Instructions:

1. Mash avocado and spread it on toasted whole-grain bread.

2. Top with tomato slices, crumbled feta cheese, olive oil, and fresh basil.

Breakfast:

6. *Mediterranean Breakfast Burrito*

Ingredients:

* Whole-grain tortilla

* Scrambled eggs

* Spinach or arugula

* Roasted red peppers (sliced)

* Feta cheese

* Kalamata olives (sliced)

Instructions:

1. Fill a tortilla with scrambled eggs, spinach or arugula, roasted red peppers, crumbled feta cheese, and sliced olives.

2. Roll it up and enjoy a nutritious breakfast on the go.

7. *Mediterranean Chia Pudding*

Ingredients:

* Chia seeds

* Greek yogurt

* Fresh berries

* Honey

* Almonds (chopped)

Instructions:

1. Mix chia seeds with Greek yogurt and let it sit in the fridge overnight.

2. In the morning, top with fresh berries, honey, and chopped almonds.

Breakfast:

8. *Mediterranean Breakfast Couscous*

Ingredients:

* Whole wheat couscous

* Chopped dried apricots

* Chopped almonds

* Greek yogurt

* Honey

* Ground cinnamon

Instructions:

1. Cook couscous in line with package instructions.

2. Mix in chopped dried apricots and almonds.

3. Top with Greek yogurt, honey, and a sprinkle of ground cinnamon.

9. *Mediterranean Oatmeal Bowl*

Ingredients:

* Rolled oats

* Chopped dates

* Sliced bananas

* Chopped pistachios

* Drizzle of tahini

Instructions:

1. Prepare oats with water or milk.

2. Top with chopped dates, sliced bananas, chopped pistachios, and a drizzle of tahini.

Breakfast:

10. ***Mediterranean Breakfast Wrap***

Ingredients:

* Whole-grain wrap

* Scrambled eggs

* Sliced avocado

* Sliced tomatoes

* Feta cheese

* Fresh basil leaves

Instructions:

1. Fill a whole-grain wrap with scrambled eggs, avocado slices, tomato slices, crumbled feta cheese, and fresh basil leaves.

2. Roll it up and enjoy a savory breakfast.

11. ***Mediterranean Chia Seed Pudding Parfait***

Ingredients:

* Chia seeds

* Greek yogurt

* Fresh mixed berries

* Honey

* Chopped pistachios

Instructions:

1. Mix chia seeds with Greek yogurt and refrigerate overnight.

2. In the morning, layer the chia seed pudding with fresh berries, honey, and chopped pistachios in a glass.

Breakfast:

12. *Mediterranean Omelette with Spinach and Feta*

Ingredients:

* Eggs

* Fresh spinach

* Crumbled feta cheese

* Sliced black olives

* Extra-virgin olive oil

Instructions:

1. Sauté fresh spinach in olive oil until wilted.

2. Pour beaten eggs over the spinach.

3. Add crumbled feta cheese and sliced black olives.

4. Cook until the eggs are set, then fold and serve.

13. *Mediterranean Overnight Oats*

Ingredients:

* Rolled oats

* Greek yogurt

* Sliced banana

* Chopped dates

* Chopped pistachios

* Honey

Instructions:

1. Mix rolled oats with Greek yogurt and refrigerate overnight.

2. In the morning, top with sliced banana, chopped dates, chopped pistachios, and a drizzle of honey.

Breakfast:

14. ***Mediterranean Breakfast Scramble***

Ingredients:

* Eggs

* Chopped spinach

* Diced tomatoes

* Chopped red bell pepper

* Crumbled feta cheese

* Fresh basil leaves (chopped)

Instructions:

1. Scramble eggs in a pan and add chopped spinach, diced tomatoes, red bell pepper, and crumbled feta cheese.

2. Garnish with fresh basil leaves before serving.

15. *Mediterranean Chia Yogurt Parfait*

Ingredients:

* Greek yogurt

* Chia seeds

* Sliced kiwi

* Pomegranate seeds

* Drizzle of honey

Instructions:

1. Mix chia seeds with Greek yogurt and let it sit in the fridge.

2. Layer the chia yogurt with sliced kiwi, pomegranate seeds, and a drizzle of honey in a glass.

1. ***Mediterranean Chickpea Salad***

Ingredients:

   * Canned chickpeas (rinsed and drained)

   * Cherry tomatoes (halved)

   * Cucumber (diced)

   * Red onion (thinly sliced)

   * Kalamata olives (pitted)

   * Feta cheese (crumbled, optional)

   * Fresh parsley (chopped)

   * Extra-virgin olive oil

   * Lemon juice

   * Salt and pepper to taste

Instructions:

1. In a large bowl, combine chickpeas, cherry tomatoes, cucumber, red onion, and Kalamata olives.

2. Drizzle with extra-virgin olive oil and lemon juice.

3. Season with salt and pepper, then toss well.

4. Top with crumbled feta cheese (if desired) and fresh parsley.

5. Serve as a healthy and satisfying salad.

2. *Mediterranean Quinoa Salad*

Ingredients:

* Cooked quinoa

* Cherry tomatoes (halved)

* Cucumber (diced)

* Red onion (chopped)

* Feta cheese

* Kalamata olives

* Fresh mint (chopped)

* Lemon vinaigrette (mixture of lemon juice and olive oil)

Instructions:

1. Combine cooked quinoa with vegetables, feta, olives, and mint.

2. Drizzle with lemon vinaigrette and toss well.

3. *Mediterranean Lentil Soup*

Ingredients:

   * Lentils

   * Carrots (diced)

   * Celery (chopped)

   * Onion (chopped)

   * Garlic (minced)

   * Vegetable broth

   * Cumin and coriander (for seasoning)

   * Fresh lemon juice

Instructions:

   1. Sauté vegetables and garlic in olive oil.

   2. Add lentils, vegetable broth, and seasonings. Simmer until lentils are tender.

   3. Finish with a squeeze of fresh lemon juice.

4. *Mediterranean Tuna Salad*

Ingredients:

   * Canned tuna (in water, drained)

   * Cucumbers (diced)

   * Red onion (chopped)

   * Cherry tomatoes (halved)

* Kalamata olives

* Olive oil and lemon juice (for dressing)

* Fresh dill (chopped)

Instructions:

1. Mix tuna, cucumbers, red onion, tomatoes, and olives in a bowl.

2. Drizzle with olive oil and lemon juice, then sprinkle with fresh dill.

5. **Mediterranean Stuffed Pita**

Ingredients:

* Whole-grain pita bread

* Hummus

* Sliced roasted red peppers

* Sliced cucumbers

* Baby spinach leaves

* Sliced grilled chicken (optional)

Instructions:

1. Spread hummus inside the pita pockets.

2. Stuff with roasted red peppers, cucumbers, spinach, and grilled chicken (if desired).

6. ***Mediterranean Roasted Vegetable Wrap***

Ingredients:

* Whole-grain wrap

* Roasted vegetables (e.g., eggplant, zucchini, and bell peppers)

* Hummus

* Fresh basil leaves

Instructions:

1. Spread hummus on the wrap.

2. Add roasted vegetables and fresh basil.

3. Roll it up and enjoy a flavorful and healthy wrap.

8. ***Mediterranean Lentil and Quinoa Bowl***

Ingredients:

* Cooked lentils

* Cooked quinoa

* Cherry tomatoes (halved)

* Cucumber (diced)

* Red onion (chopped)

* Feta cheese

* Lemon-tahini dressing

Instructions:

1. Combine cooked lentils and quinoa in a bowl.

2. Add cherry tomatoes, cucumber, red onion, and crumbled feta cheese.

3. Drizzle with lemon-tahini dressing for added flavor.

9. *Mediterranean Tabbouleh Salad*

Ingredients:

* Bulgur wheat

* Fresh parsley (chopped)

* Tomatoes (diced)

* Cucumber (diced)

* Red onion (finely chopped)

* Fresh mint leaves (chopped)

* Lemon juice and olive oil (to dress)

Instructions:

1. Combine cooked bulgur with vegetables and herbs.

2. Dress with lemon juice and olive oil for a refreshing salad.

10. *Mediterranean Pita Pizza*

Ingredients:

* Whole-grain pita bread

* Tomato sauce

* Sliced black olives

* Sliced artichoke hearts

* Sliced cherry tomatoes

* Crumbled goat cheese

Instructions:

1. Spread tomato sauce on pita bread.

2. Add olives, artichoke hearts, cherry tomatoes, and goat cheese.

3. Bake until cheese is melted and toppings are heated through.

11. ***Mediterranean Falafel Bowl***

Ingredients:

* Homemade or store-bought falafel

* Quinoa or bulgur wheat

* Sliced cucumbers

* Cherry tomatoes (halved)

* Tzatziki sauce

* Fresh cilantro leaves

* Instructions:

1. Prepare falafel and quinoa or bulgur wheat.

2. Assemble a bowl with falafel, grains, cucumbers, tomatoes, a drizzle of tzatziki sauce, and fresh cilantro leaves.

12. *Mediterranean Spinach and Feta Stuffed Chicken Breast*

Ingredients:

* Boneless, skinless chicken breasts

* Fresh spinach leaves

* Crumbled feta cheese

* Lemon zest

* Garlic (minced)

Instructions:

1. Create a hollow space in each chicken breast.

2. Stuff with fresh spinach, crumbled feta, lemon zest, and minced garlic.

3. Bake until the chicken is well cooked.

13. *Mediterranean Orzo Salad*

Ingredients:

* Cooked orzo pasta

* Cherry tomatoes (halved)

* Kalamata olives (pitted and sliced)

* Red onion (finely chopped)

* Fresh basil leaves (chopped)

* Balsamic vinaigrette dressing

Instructions:

1. Toss cooked orzo pasta with cherry tomatoes, Kalamata olives, red onion, and fresh basil.

2. Drizzle with balsamic vinaigrette dressing.

14. ***Mediterranean Veggie Wrap***

* Ingredients:

   * Whole-grain wrap

   * Hummus

   * Sliced roasted red peppers

   * Sliced cucumbers

   * Baby spinach leaves

   * Sliced black olives

Instructions:

1. Spread hummus on a whole-grain wrap.

2. Add roasted red peppers, cucumbers, baby spinach leaves, and sliced black olives.

3. Roll it up and enjoy a fresh and satisfying wrap.

15. *Mediterranean White Bean Salad*

Ingredients:

* Canned cannellini beans, thoroughly rinsed and drained.

* Cherry tomatoes (halved)

* Chopped cucumber

* Red onion (chopped)

* Fresh parsley (chopped)

* Lemon-tahini dressing

Instructions:

1. Combine cannellini beans, cherry tomatoes, cucumber, red onion, and fresh parsley.

2. Dress with lemon-tahini dressing for a protein-packed salad.

16. *Mediterranean Lentil and Vegetable Soup*

Ingredients:

* Green or brown lentils

* Carrots (sliced)

* Celery (chopped)

* Onion (chopped)

* Garlic (minced)

* Vegetable broth

* Fresh lemon juice

Instructions:

1. Sauté onions, garlic, carrots, and celery in olive oil.

2. Add lentils, vegetable broth, and simmer until lentils and vegetables are tender.

3. Finish with a squeeze of fresh lemon juice.

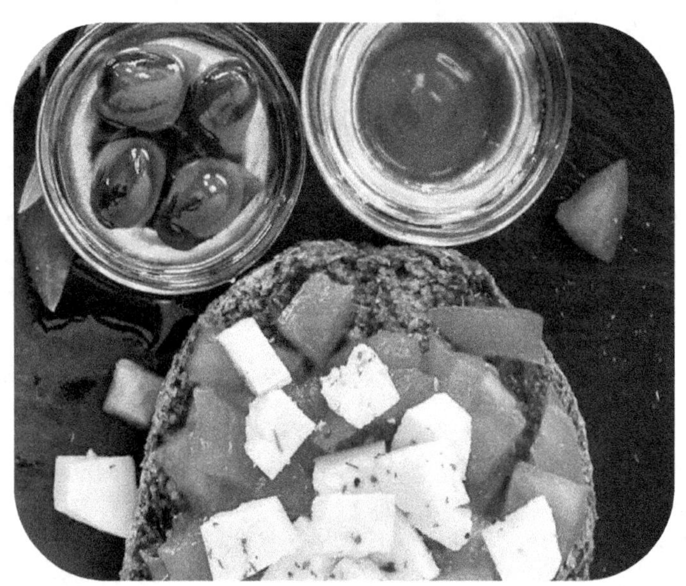

1. *Mediterranean Baked Salmon*

Ingredients:

* Salmon fillet

* Extra-virgin olive oil

* Lemon juice

* Garlic (minced)

* Fresh herbs (e.g., rosemary, thyme, or oregano)

* Cherry tomatoes

* Kalamata olives

* Salt and pepper to taste

Instructions:

1. Preheat the oven to about 375°F (190°C).

2. on a baking sheet lined with parchment paper Place the salmon fillet

3. In a small bowl, mix olive oil, lemon juice, minced garlic, and chopped fresh herbs.

4. Drizzle the mixture over the salmon and season with salt and pepper.

5. Add cherry tomatoes and Kalamata olives around the salmon.

6. Bake for about 15-20 minutes or until the salmon flakes easily with a fork.

7. Serve with a side of whole-grain couscous or quinoa and steamed vegetables.

2. *Mediterranean Stuffed Bell Peppers*

Ingredients:

* Bell peppers (red, yellow, or green)

* Lean ground turkey or chicken

* Quinoa

* Tomatoes (diced)

* Feta cheese

* Fresh herbs (such as parsley or dill)

Instructions:

1. Cut the tops off bell peppers and remove seeds.

2. Mix cooked quinoa, browned ground meat, diced tomatoes, feta, and herbs.

3. Stuff peppers with the mixture and bake until peppers are tender.

3. *Mediterranean Grilled Chicken with Tzatziki Sauce*

Ingredients:

* Chicken breasts or thighs

* Greek yogurt-based tzatziki sauce

* Lemon juice

* Garlic (minced)

* Herbs (like oregano and thyme)

Instructions:

1. Marinate chicken in a mixture of yogurt, lemon juice, garlic, and herbs.

2. Grill until fully cooked and serve with tzatziki sauce.

4. **Mediterranean Veggie and Chickpea Curry**

Ingredients:

* Chickpeas (canned or cooked)

* Eggplant (diced)

* Zucchini (sliced)

* Bell peppers (sliced)

* Tomatoes (diced)

* Coconut milk

* Curry spices (e.g., cumin, turmeric, and coriander)

* Fresh cilantro (chopped)

Instructions:

1. Sauté vegetables in olive oil until tender.

2. Add chickpeas, tomatoes, coconut milk, and curry spices.

3. Simmer until flavors meld and garnish with fresh cilantro.

5. ***Mediterranean Stuffed Portobello Mushrooms***

Ingredients:

* Portobello mushrooms (stems removed)

* Quinoa or couscous

* Spinach (sautéed)

* Sundried tomatoes (chopped)

* Feta cheese

* Instructions:

1. Roast or grill the mushrooms.

2. Stuff with cooked quinoa or couscous mixed with sautéed spinach, sundried tomatoes, and crumbled feta cheese.

6. ***Mediterranean Stuffed Acorn Squash***

Ingredients:

* Acorn squash (halved and roasted)

* Ground turkey or chickpeas (cooked)

* Quinoa

* Diced tomatoes

* Spinach (sautéed)

* Pine nuts (toasted)

Instructions:

1. Bake the halves of acorn squash until they become soft.

2. Fill with a mixture of cooked ground turkey or chickpeas, quinoa, diced tomatoes, sautéed spinach, and toasted pine nuts.

7. *Mediterranean Baked Eggplant Parmesan*

Ingredients:

* Sliced eggplant (breaded and baked)

* Marinara sauce

* Mozzarella cheese (part-skim)

* Fresh basil leaves

Instructions:

1. Layer baked eggplant slices with marinara sauce and mozzarella cheese.

2. Bake until cheese is melted and bubbly.

3. Garnish with fresh basil leaves

8. ***Mediterranean Lentil Stew***

Ingredients:

   * Green or brown lentils

   * Carrots (sliced)

   * Celery (chopped)

   * Onion (chopped)

   * Garlic (minced)

   * Vegetable broth

   * Cumin and coriander (for seasoning)

Instructions:

   1. Sauté onions, garlic, carrots, and celery in olive oil.

   2. Add lentils, vegetable broth, and seasonings.

   3. Simmer until lentils and vegetables are tender.

9. ***Mediterranean Grilled Shrimp Skewers***

Ingredients:

   * Shrimp (peeled and deveined)

   * Cherry tomatoes

   * Red bell pepper (sliced)

   * Red onion (sliced)

   * Lemon juice and olive oil (for marinade)

Instructions:

1. Marinate shrimp in a mixture of lemon juice and olive oil.

2. Thread shrimp, cherry tomatoes, red bell pepper, and red onion onto skewers.

3. Grill until shrimp are pink and cooked through.

10. ***Mediterranean Quinoa-Stuffed Bell Peppers***

Ingredients:

* Bell peppers (red, yellow, or green)

* Cooked quinoa

* Chickpeas (cooked)

* Chopped tomatoes

* Chopped fresh parsley

* Lemon juice and olive oil (for drizzling)

Instructions:

1. Cut the tops off bell peppers and remove seeds.

2. Stuff with a mixture of cooked quinoa, chickpeas, chopped tomatoes, and fresh parsley.

3. Drizzle with lemon juice and olive oil, then bake until peppers are tender.

11. ***Mediterranean Grilled Vegetable Skewers***

Ingredients:

* Assorted vegetables (e.g., zucchini, cherry tomatoes, mushrooms, and red onion)

* Olive oil and balsamic vinegar marinade

* Fresh thyme leaves

Instructions:

1. Thread vegetables onto skewers.

2. Marinate in olive oil and balsamic vinegar, then grill until tender.

3. Sprinkle with fresh thyme leaves before serving.

Dinner:

12. ***Mediterranean Spaghetti Squash with Pesto***

Ingredients:

* Roasted spaghetti squash

* Homemade or store-bought pesto sauce

* Cherry tomatoes (halved)

* Pine nuts (toasted)

Instructions:

1. Scrape the flesh of roasted spaghetti squash into "noodles."

2. Toss with pesto sauce, cherry tomatoes, and toasted pine nuts.

13. *Mediterranean Baked Cod*

Ingredients:

* Cod fillets

* Sliced black olives

* Chopped sun-dried tomatoes

* Fresh oregano leaves

* Lemon slices

Instructions:

1. Place cod fillets in a baking dish.

2. Top with sliced olives, sun-dried tomatoes, fresh oregano leaves, and lemon slices.

3. Bake until the fish flakes easily.

Dinner:

14. *Mediterranean Quinoa-Stuffed Acorn Squash*

Ingredients:

* Acorn squash (halved and roasted)

* Cooked quinoa

* Chopped dried apricots

* Toasted pine nuts

* Fresh mint leaves (chopped)

Instructions:

1. Bake the halves of acorn squash until they become soft..

2. Fill with a mixture of cooked quinoa, chopped dried apricots, toasted pine nuts, and chopped fresh mint.

15. ***Mediterranean Baked Zucchini Boats***

Ingredients:

* Zucchini (halved and hollowed)

* Ground turkey or plant-based protein

* Chopped tomatoes

* Crumbled feta cheese

* Fresh oregano leaves

Instructions:

1. Brown ground turkey or plant-based protein.

2. Mix with chopped tomatoes and crumbled feta cheese.

3. Stuff zucchini halves with the mixture and bake until zucchini is tender.

1. ***Mediterranean Hummus with Veggie Sticks***

Ingredients:

* Hummus (store-bought or homemade)

* Carrot sticks

* Cucumber slices

* Bell pepper strips (red or yellow)

Instructions:

1. Arrange the vegetable sticks on a plate.

2. Serve with a bowl of hummus for dipping.

3. This snack provides protein, fiber, and essential nutrients.

2. ***Mediterranean Antipasto Platter***

Ingredients:

* Assorted olives

* Sliced prosciutto or lean ham

* Sliced cheese (like mozzarella or provolone)

* Cherry tomatoes

* Whole-grain crackers

Instructions:

1. Arrange olives, prosciutto, cheese, and tomatoes on a platter.

2. Serve with whole-grain crackers for a satisfying snack.

3. **Greek Yogurt with Honey and Walnuts**

Ingredients:

* Greek yogurt

* Honey

* Chopped walnuts

Instructions:

1. Top Greek yogurt with a drizzle of honey and chopped walnuts for a quick and nutritious snack.

4. **Mediterranean Cucumber Cups**

Ingredients:

* Cucumber slices (thick)

* Tzatziki sauce

* Sliced black olives

* Cherry tomatoes (halved)

Instructions:

1. Scoop out some of the flesh from cucumber slices to create "cups."

2. Fill with tzatziki sauce, olives, and cherry tomato halves.

5. *Mediterranean Fruit Salad*

Ingredients:

* Mixed fresh fruits (e.g., oranges, grapes, and melon)

* Fresh mint leaves (chopped)

* A drizzle of honey

Instructions:

1. Combine fresh fruits in a bowl.

2. Garnish with chopped mint leaves and a drizzle of honey.

6. *Mediterranean Cucumber and Tomato Salad*

Ingredients:

* Cucumber (sliced)

* Cherry tomatoes (halved)

* Red onion (thinly sliced)

* Fresh dill (chopped)

* Red wine vinegar and olive oil (for dressing)

Instructions:

1. Combine cucumber, tomatoes, red onion, and fresh dill in a bowl.

2. Dress with a mixture of red wine vinegar and olive oil.

7. ***Mediterranean Rice Cakes***

Ingredients:

* Whole-grain rice cakes

* Hummus

* Sliced cucumber

* Sliced radishes

* Sprouts or microgreens

Instructions:

1. Spread hummus on rice cakes.

2. Top with cucumber slices, radishes, and sprouts for a crunchy and satisfying snack.

8. ***Mediterranean Trail Mix***

Ingredients:

* Almonds

* Walnuts

* Dried figs (chopped)

* Dried apricots (chopped)

* Dark chocolate chunks

Instructions:

1. Mix almonds, walnuts, dried figs, dried apricots, and dark chocolate chunks for a satisfying and nutritious trail mix.

9. *Mediterranean Cottage Cheese*

Ingredients:

* Low-fat cottage cheese

* Sliced fresh peaches

* Drizzle of honey

* Sliced almonds

Instructions:

1. Top cottage cheese with sliced peaches, a drizzle of honey, and sliced almonds for a protein-packed snack.

10. *Mediterranean Guacamole with Veggie Sticks*

Ingredients:

* Guacamole (homemade or store-bought)

* Carrot sticks

* Celery sticks

* Bell pepper strips

Instructions:

1. Serve guacamole with an assortment of veggie sticks for a nutritious and creamy snack.

11. *Mediterranean Greek-Style Yogurt with Berries and Almonds*

Ingredients:

* Greek-style yogurt

* Mixed berries

* Slivered almonds

* Drizzle of honey

Instructions:

1. Top Greek-style yogurt with mixed berries, slivered almonds, and a drizzle of honey for a protein-rich snack.

12. *Mediterranean Rice Cakes with Tzatziki*

Ingredients:

* Brown rice cakes

* Tzatziki sauce

* Sliced cucumber

* Fresh dill (chopped)

Instructions:

1. Spread tzatziki sauce on brown rice cakes.

2. Top with sliced cucumber and a sprinkle of fresh dill for a light and refreshing snack.

13. *Mediterranean Mixed Nuts*

Ingredients:

* Assorted mixed nuts (e.g., almonds, walnuts, and pistachios)

* Dried cherries or cranberries

* Cinnamon

* Instructions:

1. Mix assorted mixed nuts with dried cherries or cranberries.

2. Sprinkle with a pinch of cinnamon for a satisfying and nutritious snack.

14. *Mediterranean Cucumber Cups with Tuna Salad*

Ingredients:

* Cucumber slices (thick)

* Tuna salad (canned tuna mixed with Greek yogurt, lemon juice, and herbs)

* Cherry tomatoes (halved)

Instructions:

1. Use cucumber slices as cups to hold tuna salad.

2. Garnish with halved cherry tomatoes.

15. *Mediterranean Frozen Yogurt Bark*

Ingredients:

* Greek yogurt

* Mixed berries

* Chopped almonds

* Drizzle of honey

Instructions:

1. Spread Greek yogurt on a baking sheet.

2. Top with mixed berries, chopped almonds, and a drizzle of honey.

3. Freeze until firm, then break into pieces for a cool and nutritious snack.

In the final pages of "The Mediterranean Diet Cookbook for Pregnant Women," we have embarked on a culinary journey that is as nourishing for the body as it is for the soul.

We've explored the rich tapestry of flavors and traditions that the Mediterranean diet has to offer, and we've harnessed its bountiful benefits to support and celebrate the incredible journey of pregnancy.

As we close this chapter, I hope you are armed with not just delectable recipes, but with a deep understanding of the profound connection between what we eat and the precious life growing within.

The Mediterranean diet has not only provided us with a palette of delicious and diverse dishes but also a profound lesson in embracing nature's bounty and savoring the simplest, most wholesome ingredients.

But beyond the recipes and ingredients, this cookbook has been about the celebration of life. The nine-month journey of pregnancy is a transformative and awe-inspiring period in a woman's life, and what better way to honor this experience than by nourishing both body and spirit with the time-honored wisdom of the Mediterranean diet?

I hope that this book has not only tantalized your taste buds but also empowered you with the knowledge to make informed and healthful choices for yourself and your growing baby.

As you flip through these pages one last time, remember that the Mediterranean diet is not just a dietary plan; it's a way of life that champions balance, vitality, and the joy of savoring each bite.

May your pregnancy be filled with vibrant health, abundant joy, and unforgettable meals shared with loved ones. Here's to a radiant and delicious journey into motherhood, guided by the timeless wisdom of the Mediterranean diet.

As you savor the recipes within, I hope you also savor the incredible adventure that is pregnancy. Thank you for inviting these culinary traditions into your home, your heart, and your family.

Wishing you a future filled with love, good health, and the shared delights of the Mediterranean table. Bon appétit and blessings on this beautiful chapter of your life!

MARRIES E. LLOYD

AUTHOR

Thank you for choosing this book, if you feel this book is valuable, kindly consider leaving us a review on Amazon. Your feedback is critical to me and others looking for help related to the same book.